THE MEN'S PREVENTIVE HEALTH GUIDE

WHAT TO CHECK, WHEN TO CHECK IT, AND WHY IT MATTERS

LEO MOORE
MD, MSHPM

THE MEN'S PREVENTIVE HEALTH GUIDE

This book is intended solely as a reference, not a medical manual. The information provided is designed to help you make informed decisions about your health. It is not a substitute for any treatment, screening, or immunization prescribed or recommended by your doctor. If you suspect you have a medical problem, please seek medical assistance.

© 2025 by Moore Innovations, LLC

All rights reserved. No part of this publication may be reproduced or transmitted in any form or by any means, electronic or mechanical, including photocopying, recording, or any other information storage and retrieval system, without the publisher's permission.

This book may be purchased for business or promotional use or for special sales. For information, please get in touch with us at drleomoore.com.

Cover design by Oladimeji Basit. Cover photography by Jacquelyn Soria.

Library of Congress Cataloging-in-Publication Data is on file.
ISBN-13 979-8-9986648-0-9 (paperback)
ISBN-13 979-8-9986648-1-6 (e-book)

Printed in the United States of America

*For Anthony, Lannie, Robert, Warner,
and all the men who departed this Earth too soon
due to preventable health conditions.*

CONTENTS

Foreword	ix
How to Use This Guide	xi
1. Men in Their 20s	1
2. Men in Their 30s	11
3. Men in Their 40s	23
4. Men in Their 50s	35
5. Men in Their 60s	47
6. Men 70 and Older	59
7. Special Populations	69
Appendix	79
Glossary of Acronyms & Definitions	81
Thank You	85
Bibliography	87

FOREWORD

As an internal medicine physician, I've had the privilege of caring for men at every stage of life, from young guys just starting out, to fathers juggling family and work, to older men navigating new chapters in retirement. However, across all those ages, one thing remains constant: preventive care saves lives, but too many men fail to take advantage of it.

Sometimes, it's because life gets in the way. Sometimes, it's because no one explained what's important to check for and when. And other times, it's because men weren't taught to prioritize their health. That's why I created this guide.

This isn't about scaring you into tests or overwhelming you with medical jargon. It's about breaking down what you need to know by age in a practical, straightforward way grounded in the best available evidence. You'll find trusted guidelines, honest explanations, checklists, and concise recommendations to help you take charge of your health, all in one place.

FOREWORD

Whether you're reading this for yourself, a partner, or someone you care about, I hope it helps you feel more confident navigating your health journey. The goal isn't perfection, it's awareness, action, and longevity.

Let's get started.

HOW TO USE THIS GUIDE

This guide is designed to help you stay healthy at every stage of life by focusing on evidence-based screenings and immunizations for men—organized by age group and tailored to real-world needs. It is intended to be a conversation starter for you and your doctor, ensuring that you have baseline knowledge about the most common screenings and immunizations. Prevention is power and this guide puts the power in your hands.

Each Chapter Covers:

- Screening recommendations for common conditions like heart disease, diabetes, and cancer
- Vaccination schedules to protect against preventable infections
- Recommendations for men with specific conditions, backgrounds, or life experiences

- Citations and guidelines from trusted sources like the U.S. Preventive Services Task Force (USPSTF), Centers for Disease Control and Prevention (CDC), and specialty societies

Chapters Are Organized by Decade:

Each chapter includes updated medical guidance for men in their 20s, 70s, and beyond.

How to Get the Most Out of This Book:

- Jump to your age group to see what applies to you now
- Learn what's coming next so you can prepare for future milestones
- Take the book with you to your doctor's visits and use the checklists at the end of each chapter to ensure that you have all the recommended screenings and immunizations completed
- Discuss screening and treatment options with your doctor
- Bookmark or print the checklists for quick access to screening timelines and vaccine schedules

Throughout the book you will see the ☞ icon, which signifies additional notes about a topic. The first example is below:

☞ No two individuals have identical health needs. This guide offers general recommendations based on scientific guidelines but is not a substitute for personalized care from a doctor or licensed healthcare provider. Always consult your doctor or other healthcare provider before deciding about screenings or vaccinations.

WHY PREVENTIVE HEALTH MATTERS

Let's be real, most men don't go to the doctor unless something feels off. I get it. You're busy. Maybe nothing feels wrong, or you've just always toughed it out, or you may associate doctor's offices and hospitals with "bad news". But here's the deal: a lot of the significant health problems that affect men, things like heart disease, diabetes, and cancer don't usually start with symptoms. They creep up quietly, sometimes for years, and by the time you feel them, they've already done damage.

Men, on average, live five to six years less than women, and men of color, particularly Black and American Indian/Alaskan Native men, live even fewer years than women. We're more likely to die from heart disease, more likely to develop serious cancers, and far more likely not to access care for mental health. That's not because our bodies are weaker, it's because we don't do our due diligence to catch things early. And when we don't catch things early, we lose the chance to fix them while they're still manageable.

This is where preventive health comes in. It's not about turning you into a doctor's office regular; it's about taking simple steps, once a year or so, that can save your life: a quick blood pressure check, a routine colon cancer screening, a yearly flu shot, and a couple of basic lab tests. These aren't massive undertakings, but they can make a huge difference.

Prevention isn't about being perfect; it's about showing up, knowing what to look for, asking the right questions, and staying a step ahead. When you invest in your health now, you're protecting your future. This is not only about living longer, but also about feeling better, moving better, and being present for the people and the things that matter most.

CHAPTER 1
MEN IN THEIR 20S

Men in their twenties often have peak physical health, but this decade is critical for building the foundation for lifelong wellness. Regular screenings and timely immunizations can help catch potential problems early and prevent disease altogether. Most screenings in this age group are simple, low-cost, and easy to access during routine checkups.

RECOMMENDED SCREENINGS

1. Blood Pressure Screening

All men should have their blood pressure checked at least once every 2 years if normal (<120/80 mmHg), or more frequently if elevated. High blood pressure is often silent and can lead to heart disease and stroke if untreated.[1]

2. Body Mass Index (BMI)

BMI should be calculated at least once annually. While it doesn't measure body fat directly, it is a valuable screening tool for obesity-related health risks.[2]

3. Mental Health Screening

Routine depression and anxiety screening is recommended, especially for those with stress, trauma, or a family history of mental illness. This can be done via simple questionnaires during a primary care visit.[3]

4. Sexually Transmitted Infection (STI) Screening

Sexually active men should be screened for HIV at least once and every 3 – 6 months if you:

- have multiple sexual partners
- inject drugs or share drug equipment
- have condomless anal sex
- have a partner who is known to be living with HIV
- exchange sex for money, housing, or other resources
- have been diagnosed with a sexually transmitted infection (STI) in the past 6 months
- are using HIV pre-exposure prophylaxis (PrEP) – medication taken by mouth or as an injection to prevent HIV infection if you are exposed.[18]

Chlamydia, gonorrhea, and syphilis testing is also advised for those with multiple partners or other factors that increase the chances of getting an STI.[4]

☞ **For men who are having anal and/or oral sex:** If you are the receiving partner during anal sex (i.e., bottom or versatile) or give oral sex (i.e. you put your mouth on their genitals) to your sexual partners, you must ask your doctor to swab your anus and mouth to detect gonorrhea and/or chlamydia. A urine test will NOT detect gonorrhea or chlamydia in the anus or mouth.

5. Testicular Self-Examination

Testicular cancer is the most common cancer in men ages 20 – 34. Some doctors recommend monthly self-checks, although the United States Preventive Services Task Force (USPSTF) states insufficient evidence supports routine screening in men who do not have symptoms. This should be a discussion between you and your doctor to determine if this will be done.[5] Instructions on how to complete a testicular self-examination can be found in the Appendix.

RECOMMENDED IMMUNIZATIONS & DOSING SCHEDULES

Vaccines play a significant role in protecting young adult men from preventable and sometimes life-threatening diseases. Based on CDC and ACIP guidelines, the following vaccines are recommended for men in their 20s.

Human Papillomavirus (HPV) Vaccine

- **What It Protects Against:**

- HPV is a common sexually transmitted infection that can lead to genital warts and several cancers, including anal, throat, and penile cancers. The 9-valent HPV vaccine protects against strains responsible for over 90% of these conditions.[6]
- **Who Should Get It:**
  - Men up to age 26 who were not previously vaccinated.
  - Can also be given to men up to age 45 if they have any of the following:
    - New or multiple sex partners
    - Men who have sex with men
    - Immunocompromised individuals, including those with HIV
    - Individuals who did not complete the vaccine series at a young age
    - History of STIs or inconsistent condom use
    - Partners with increased chance of having HPV (e.g., multiple partners or GBMSM)[6]
- **Dosing Schedule:**
  - 2 doses (if series starts before age 15):
    - Dose 1
    - Dose 2: 6 – 12 months later
  - 3 doses (if series starts at age 15 or older):
    - Dose 1
    - Dose 2: 1 – 2 months later
    - Dose 3: 6 months after the first dose[11]

Tetanus, Diphtheria, and Pertussis (Tdap) Vaccine

- **What It Protects Against:**
    - **Tetanus** – a serious bacterial infection that causes severe muscle stiffness, spasms, and can lead to death.
    - **Diphtheria** – a severe bacterial infection of the nose and throat that creates a thick, gray substance that covers the back of the throat, making breathing hard.
    - **Pertussis (whooping cough)** – a highly contagious bacterial infection that can cause violent coughing fits and is especially dangerous to infants.
- **Who Should Get It:** Adults who have never received Tdap.
- **Dosing Schedule:**
    - 1 dose of Tdap, then a booster every 10 years[7].

☞ Most men completed the initial Tdap vaccine series during childhood, but you may be due for a booster.

- **Effectiveness:**
    - **Pertussis protection**: Approximately 69 – 85% effective within the first year after vaccination.[12]
    - **Tetanus and diphtheria protection**: Nearly 100% effective after completing the whole 3-dose childhood DTaP series and Tdap booster, although immunity wanes over time.
    - **Duration**: Pertussis protection decreases

significantly after 1 – 2 years, so boosters are needed every 10 years.

Meningococcal Vaccines

- **What They Protect Against:**
    - *Meningococcal disease* can lead to meningitis, an infection in the thin layers of tissue covering the brain. This disease can also spread to the blood, causing infection throughout the body and increasing the risk of death within hours. Two types of vaccines cover different serogroups:

MenACWY (Quadrivalent) Vaccine

- **Who Should Get It:**
    - College students living in dorms
    - Military recruits
    - Those with specific health conditions (Ex, HIV)
    - Men who have sex with men during community outbreaks. *Some doctors may recommend it to prevent potential exposure in case of a future outbreak.*
- **Dosing Schedule:**
    - 1 dose, with booster every 5 years if chances of catching the disease still remain[14]
- **Effectiveness:**
    - Effectiveness against serogroups A, C, W, and Y is estimated at 80 – 85% in adolescents and young adults.[14]

- **Duration**: Immunity wanes after 5 years, so boosters are recommended for those with increased chances of being infected with the disease.

MenB Vaccine

- **Who Should Get It:**
    - Men aged 16 – 23, based on a conversation between you and your doctor
    - Those with increased vulnerability to the infection or those exposed during outbreaks
- **Dosing Schedule:**
    - Depending on which vaccine version you receive, you will need two doses given 1 month or 6 months apart.[14]
- **Effectiveness:**
    - Effectiveness against serogroup B is estimated at 78 – 83% depending on the vaccine given, the dosing schedule, and the age group.[16,17]
- **Duration**: Protection decreases within 1 – 2 years; boosters are generally not recommended unless the individual remains at high risk.

Influenza (Flu) Vaccine

- **What It Protects Against:**
    - The flu is a highly contagious respiratory illness that can cause fever, chills, fatigue, and body aches. It can also lead to serious complications, including pneumonia and hospitalization.

- **Who Should Get It:** Everyone 6 months and older should get a flu shot yearly.
- **Dosing Schedule:**
    - 1 dose annually, ideally before the start of flu season in the fall[8]
- **Effectiveness:** The vaccine reduces the risk of flu illness by 40 – 60% during years when the vaccine strains closely match circulating viruses[13]

COVID-19 Vaccine

- **What It Protects Against:**
    - COVID-19 can cause a wide range of respiratory symptoms. It may lead to severe illness, hospitalization, or death, especially in people with chronic medical conditions or a weakened immune system which increase their risk for severe illness.
- **Who Should Get It:** According to the latest CDC guidance, all adults should stay current with COVID-19 vaccination.
- **Dosing Schedule:**
    - **Primary series:** Typically two doses of an mRNA vaccine, 3 – 4 weeks apart
    - **Boosters:** Given as needed based on updated strain recommendations and personal risk[15]

Men's Health Checklist: Ages 20 - 29

Bring this list to your next checkup. Use it to ask questions and ensure you're up to date on your preventive care.

Recommended Screenings

Screening	Completed	Notes
Blood Pressure	☐	
BMI/Weight Check	☐	
Mental Health	☐	
HIV & STI	☐	
Testicular Self-Exam (optional)	☐	Discuss with doctor.

Recommended Immunizations

Immunization	Completed	Notes
HPV	☐	
Tdap (once if never received)	☐	Booster every 10 yrs.
Influenza (annually)	☐	Get every fall
Meningitis	☐	
COVID-19 (primary & booster(s))	☐	

Talk With Your Doctor About:

- Any new or ongoing symptoms
- Family history of chronic illness or cancer
- Alcohol, tobacco, or drug use
- Sexual health and STI prevention
- Sleep, stress, and mental health

CHAPTER 2
MEN IN THEIR 30S

Men in their thirties are often focused on careers, family, and building stability, but health must still be a top priority. Many chronic conditions, such as high blood pressure, diabetes, and high cholesterol, begin to develop silently during this decade. Maintaining routine health screenings and staying up to date on vaccinations can help detect issues early and prevent long-term complications.

RECOMMENDED SCREENINGS

1. Blood Pressure Screening

Men should continue having their blood pressure checked at least every 2 years if readings are normal (<120/80 mmHg) and more frequently if elevated. High blood pressure is a leading risk factor for heart attack and stroke.[1]

2. BMI and Obesity Risk

Body mass index (BMI) should be assessed annually. Obesity increases the risk of type 2 diabetes, sleep apnea, and cardiovascular disease.[2]

3. Mental Health Screening

Depression and anxiety screenings should continue, especially for men experiencing stress, family changes, or burnout. Early identification can significantly improve the quality of life.[3]

4. Sexually Transmitted Infections (STIs)

Sexually active men should be screened for HIV at least once and every 3 – 6 months if you:

- have multiple sexual partners
- inject drugs or share drug equipment
- have condomless anal sex
- have a partner who is known to be living with HIV
- exchange sex for money, housing, or other resources
- have been diagnosed with a sexually transmitted infection (STI) in the past 6 months
- are using HIV pre-exposure prophylaxis (PrEP) – medication taken by mouth or as an injection to prevent HIV infection if you are exposed.[18]

Chlamydia, gonorrhea, and syphilis testing is also advised for those with multiple partners or other factors that increase the chances of getting an STI.[4]

☞ **For men who are having anal and/or oral sex:** If you are the receiving partner during anal sex (i.e., bottom or versatile) or give oral sex (i.e. you put your mouth on their genitals) to your sexual partners, you must ask your doctor to swab your anus and mouth to detect gonorrhea and/or chlamydia. A urine test will NOT detect gonorrhea or chlamydia in the anus or mouth.

5. Lipid Panel (Cholesterol Test)

Start lipid screening at age 35 for average-risk men and earlier (age 20 – 30) for those with diabetes, obesity, or a family history of heart disease. [19]

6. Diabetes Screening

Men with a BMI ≥ 25 and at least one additional risk factor (e.g., family history, high blood pressure) should be screened starting at age 35 and every 3 years thereafter. People with the following risk factors should be screened every 12 months to catch conversion to diabetes quickly and guide lifestyle changes and medication decisions.

1. History of gestational diabetes (in men, often a family history in a female partner may signal shared lifestyle risk)
2. Prediabetes (HbA1c 5.7 – 6.4%, fasting glucose 100 –125 mg/dL)

3. Hypertension (≥140/90 mmHg or on therapy)
4. Low HDL (<35 mg/dL) or high triglycerides (>250 mg/dL)
5. History of heart disease or stroke
6. Family history – parent or sibling with diabetes
7. Black, Latino, Native American, Asian American, or Pacific Islander ethnicity
8. Sedentary lifestyle
9. Obesity or severe obesity[32]

Screening uses fasting glucose or Hemoglobin A1c tests, which are both blood tests.[20]

RECOMMENDED IMMUNIZATIONS & DOSING SCHEDULES

Vaccines play a significant role in protecting young adult men from preventable and sometimes life-threatening diseases. The following vaccines are recommended for men in their 30s, based on CDC and ACIP guidelines.

Human Papillomavirus (HPV) Vaccine

- **What It Protects Against:**
    - HPV is a common sexually transmitted infection that can lead to genital warts and several cancers, including anal, throat, and penile cancers. The 9-valent HPV vaccine protects against strains responsible for over 90% of these conditions.[6]
- **Who Should Get It:**

- Men up to age 26 who were not previously vaccinated.
- Can also be given to men up to age 45 if they have any of the following:
   - New or multiple sex partners
   - Men who have sex with men
   - Immunocompromised individuals, including those with HIV
   - Individuals who did not complete the vaccine series at a young age
   - History of STIs or inconsistent condom use
   - Partners with increased chance of having HPV (e.g., multiple partners or GBMSM)[6]
- **Dosing Schedule:**
  - 2 doses (if series starts before age 15):
    - Dose 1
    - Dose 2: 6 – 12 months later
  - 3 doses (if series starts at age 15 or older):
    - Dose 1
    - Dose 2: 1 – 2 months later
    - Dose 3: 6 months after the first dose[11]

Tetanus, Diphtheria, and Pertussis (Tdap) Vaccine

- **What It Protects Against:**
  - **Tetanus** – a serious bacterial infection that causes severe muscle stiffness, spasms, and can lead to death.
  - **Diphtheria** – a severe bacterial infection of the nose and throat that creates a thick, gray substance that

covers the back of the throat, making breathing hard.
- **Pertussis (whooping cough)** – a highly contagious bacterial infection that can cause violent coughing fits and is especially dangerous to infants.
- **Who Should Get It:** Adults who have never received Tdap.
- **Dosing Schedule:**
  - 1 dose of Tdap, then a Td or Tdap booster every 10 years[7].

☞ Most men completed the initial Tdap vaccine series during childhood, but you may be due for a booster.

- **Effectiveness:**
  - **Pertussis protection**: Approximately 69 – 85% effective within the first year after vaccination.[12]
  - **Tetanus and diphtheria protection**: Nearly 100% effective after completing the whole 3-dose childhood DTaP series and Tdap booster, although immunity wanes over time.
  - **Duration**: Pertussis protection decreases significantly after 1 – 2 years, so boosters are needed every 10 years.

Meningococcal Vaccines

- **What They Protect Against:** *Meningococcal disease* can lead to meningitis, an infection in the thin layers of tissue covering the brain. This disease can also spread to the blood, causing infection throughout the body and increasing the risk of death within hours. Two types of vaccines cover different serogroups:

MenACWY (Quadrivalent) Vaccine

- **Who Should Get It:**
    - College students living in dorms
    - Military recruits
    - Those with specific health conditions (Ex, HIV)
    - Men who have sex with men during community outbreaks. *Some doctors may recommend it to prevent potential exposure in case of a future outbreak.*
- **Dosing Schedule:**
    - 1 dose, with booster every 5 years if chances of catching the disease still remain[14]
- **Effectiveness:**
    - Effectiveness against serogroups A, C, W, and Y is estimated at 80 – 85% in adolescents and young adults.[14]
- **Duration**: Immunity wanes after 5 years, so boosters are recommended for those with increased chances of being infected with the disease.

MenB Vaccine

- **Who Should Get It:**
    - Men aged 16 – 23, based on a conversation between you and your doctor.

- Those with increased vulnerability to the infection or those exposed during outbreaks.
- **Dosing Schedule:**
    - Depending on which vaccine version you receive, you will need two doses given 1 month or 6 months apart.[14]
- **Effectiveness:**
    - Effectiveness against serogroup B is estimated at 78 – 83% depending on the vaccine given, the dosing schedule, and the age group.[16,17]
- **Duration**: Protection decreases within 1 – 2 years; boosters are generally not recommended unless the individual remains at high risk.

Influenza (Flu) Vaccine

- **What It Protects Against:**
    - The flu is a highly contagious respiratory illness that can cause fever, chills, fatigue, and body aches. It can also lead to serious complications, including pneumonia and hospitalization.
- **Who Should Get It:** Everyone 6 months and older should get a flu shot yearly.
- **Dosing Schedule:**
    - 1 dose annually, ideally before the start of flu season in the fall[8]
- **Effectiveness:** The vaccine reduces the risk of flu illness by 40 – 60% during years when the vaccine strains closely match circulating viruses.[13]

COVID-19 Vaccine

- **What It Protects Against:**
  - COVID-19 can cause a wide range of respiratory symptoms. It may lead to severe illness, hospitalization, or death, especially in people with chronic medical conditions or a weakened immune system which increase their risk for severe illness.
- **Who Should Get It:** According to the latest CDC guidance, all adults should stay current with COVID-19 vaccination.
- **Dosing Schedule:**
  - **Primary series:** Typically two doses of an mRNA vaccine, 3 – 4 weeks apart
  - **Boosters:** Given as needed based on updated strain recommendations and personal risk[15]

Men's Health Checklist: Ages 30 - 39

Bring this list to your next checkup. Use it to ask questions and ensure you're up to date on your preventive care.

Recommended Screenings

Screening	Completed	Notes
Blood Pressure	☐	
BMI/Waist Circumference	☐	
Mental Health	☐	
HIV & STI	☐	
Lipid Panel (Cholesterol)	☐	
Diabetes	☐	

Recommended Immunizations

	Completed	Notes
HPV	☐	
Tdap (once if never received)	☐	Booster every 10 yrs.
Influenza (annually)	☐	Get every fall
COVID-19 (primary & booster(s))	☐	

Talk With Your Doctor About:

- Work stress, burnout, or sleep issues
- Reproductive health or planning to have children
- Alcohol, tobacco, or drug use
- Diet, exercise, and weight goals
- Cancer risks based on your family history

CHAPTER 3
MEN IN THEIR 40S

The 40s are a time when subtle changes in health can begin to surface. It's a pivotal decade for catching risk factors early, especially for heart disease, diabetes, and certain cancers. Men in this age group should start making shared decisions with their doctor about cancer screenings and maintain a strong foundation of preventive care.

RECOMMENDED SCREENINGS

1. Blood Pressure

Continue screening at least every 2 years (annually if elevated). High blood pressure is a significant risk factor for stroke, heart disease, and kidney problems.[1]

2. Body Mass Index (BMI) and Metabolic Risk

Annual measurement of weight, height, and BMI helps monitor risk for obesity-related conditions.[2]

3. Lipid Panel (Cholesterol)

Men should have a fasting or non-fasting cholesterol panel every 4 – 6 years, or more often if they have high risk (family history, diabetes, hypertension).[19]

4. Diabetes Screening

Men aged 40 – 70 who are overweight or obese should be screened for type 2 diabetes every 3 years using fasting glucose or Hemoglobin A1c, which are both blood tests.[20] People with the following risk factors should be screened every 12 months to catch conversion to diabetes quickly and guide lifestyle changes and medication decisions:

1. History of gestational diabetes (in men, often a family history in a female partner may signal shared lifestyle risk)
2. Prediabetes (HbA1c 5.7 – 6.4%, fasting glucose 100 – 125 mg/dL)
3. Hypertension (≥140/90 mmHg or on therapy)
4. Low HDL (<35 mg/dL) or high triglycerides (>250 mg/dL)
5. History of heart disease or stroke
6. Family history – parent or sibling with diabetes

7. Black, Latino, Native American, Asian American, or Pacific Islander ethnicity
8. Sedentary lifestyle
9. Obesity or severe obesity[32]

5. Mental Health and Substance Use

Continue regular screenings for depression, anxiety, and alcohol misuse during routine visits.[3]

6. Colorectal Cancer Screening

Routine screening begins at age 45 for average-risk adults, using one of the following:

- Stool-based tests (e.g., FIT annually)
- Colonoscopy every 10 years[21]

7. Prostate Cancer Screening

Prostate cancer screening should begin between ages 40 and 45 for Black men due to the higher incidence of prostate cancer and rate of Black men dying from it.[32] For men of other races and ethnicities, decision-making is encouraged starting around age 45 – 50, especially for those with a family history. Screening includes a PSA (prostate-specific antigen) blood test and a digital rectal exam optionally.[22]

8. Eye and Vision Exam

At least once in your 40s, or more frequently if you have diabetes, high blood pressure, or vision issues.[23]

9. Sexually Transmitted Infections (STIs)

Sexually active men should be screened for HIV at least once and every 3 – 6 months if you:

- have multiple sexual partners
- inject drugs or share drug equipment
- have condomless anal sex
- have a partner who is known to be living with HIV
- exchange sex for money, housing, or other resources
- have been diagnosed with a sexually transmitted infection (STI) in the past 6 months
- are using HIV pre-exposure prophylaxis (PrEP) – medication taken by mouth or as an injection to prevent HIV infection if you are exposed.[18]

Chlamydia, gonorrhea, and syphilis testing is also advised for those with multiple partners or other factors that increase the chances of getting and STI.[4]

☞ **For men who are having anal and/or oral sex:** If you are the receiving partner during anal sex (i.e., bottom or versatile) or give oral sex (i.e. you put your mouth on their genitals) to your sexual partners, you must ask your doctor to swab your anus and mouth to detect gonorrhea and/or chlamydia. A urine test will **NOT** detect gonorrhea or chlamydia in the anus or mouth.

RECOMMENDED IMMUNIZATIONS & DOSING SCHEDULES

Men in their 40s continue many of the same vaccines from earlier years but should be mindful of staying current with boosters. Here's a breakdown of the recommended immunizations with full details.

Human Papillomavirus (HPV) Vaccine

- **What It Protects Against:**
    - HPV is a common sexually transmitted infection that can lead to genital warts and several cancers, including anal, throat, and penile cancers. The 9-valent HPV vaccine protects against strains responsible for over 90% of these conditions.[6]
- **Who Should Get It:**
    - Men up to age 26 who were not previously vaccinated.
    - Can also be given to men up to age 45 if they have any of the following:
        - New or multiple sex partners
        - Men who have sex with men
        - Immunocompromised individuals, including those with HIV
        - Individuals who did not complete the vaccine series at a young age

- History of STIs or inconsistent condom use
- Partners with increased chance of having HPV (e.g., multiple partners or GBMSM)[6]
- **Dosing Schedule:**
  - 2 doses (if series starts before age 15):
    - Dose 1
    - Dose 2: 6 – 12 months later
  - 3 doses (if series starts at age 15 or older):
    - Dose 1
    - Dose 2: 1 – 2 months later
    - Dose 3: 6 months after the first dose[11]

Tetanus, Diphtheria, and Pertussis (Tdap) Vaccine

- **What It Protects Against:**
  - **Tetanus** – a serious bacterial infection that causes severe muscle stiffness, spasms, and can lead to death.
  - **Diphtheria** – a severe bacterial infection of the nose and throat that creates a thick, gray substance that covers the back of the throat, making breathing hard.
  - **Pertussis (whooping cough)** – a highly contagious bacterial infection that can cause violent coughing fits and is especially dangerous to infants.
- **Who Should Get It:** Adults who have never received Tdap.
- **Dosing Schedule:**
  - 1 dose of Tdap, then a Td or Tdap booster every 10 years[7].

☞ Most men completed the initial Tdap vaccine series during childhood, but you may be due for a booster.

- **Effectiveness:**
    - **Pertussis protection**: Approximately 69 – 85% effective within the first year after vaccination.[12]
    - **Tetanus and diphtheria protection**: Nearly 100% effective after completing the whole 3-dose childhood DTaP series and Tdap booster, although immunity wanes over time.
    - **Duration**: Pertussis protection decreases significantly after 1 – 2 years, so boosters are needed every 10 years.

Meningococcal Vaccines

- **What They Protect Against:**
    - *Meningococcal disease* can lead to meningitis, an infection in the thin layers of tissue covering the brain. This disease can also spread to the blood, causing infection throughout the body and increasing the risk of death within hours. Two types of vaccines cover different serogroups:

MenACWY (Quadrivalent) Vaccine

- **Who Should Get It:**
    - College students living in dorms
    - Military recruits
    - Those with specific health conditions (Ex, HIV)

- Men who have sex with men during community outbreaks. *Some doctors may recommend it to prevent potential exposure in case of a future outbreak.*
- **Dosing Schedule:**
  - 1 dose, with booster every 5 years if chances of catching the disease still remain[14]
- **Effectiveness:**
  - Effectiveness against serogroups A, C, W, and Y is estimated at 80 – 85% in adolescents and young adults.[14]
- **Duration**: Immunity wanes after 5 years, so boosters are recommended for those with increased chances of being infected with the disease.

MenB Vaccine

- **Who Should Get It:**
  - Men aged 16 – 23, based on a conversation between you and your doctor.
  - Those with increased vulnerability to the infection or those exposed during outbreaks.
- **Dosing Schedule:**
  - Depending on which vaccine version you receive, you will need two doses given 1 month or 6 months apart.[14]
- **Effectiveness:**
  - Effectiveness against serogroup B is estimated at 78 – 83% depending on the vaccine given, the dosing schedule, and the age group.[16,17]

- **Duration**: Protection decreases within 1 – 2 years; boosters are generally not recommended unless the individual remains at high risk.

Influenza (Flu) Vaccine

- **What It Protects Against:**
    - The flu is a highly contagious respiratory illness that can cause fever, chills, fatigue, and body aches. It can also lead to serious complications, including pneumonia and hospitalization.
- **Who Should Get It:** Everyone 6 months and older should get a flu shot yearly.
- **Dosing Schedule:**
    - 1 dose annually, ideally before the start of flu season in the fall[8]
- **Effectiveness:** The vaccine reduces the risk of flu illness by 40 – 60% during years when the vaccine strains closely match circulating viruses.[13]

COVID-19 Vaccine

- **What It Protects Against:**
    - COVID-19 can cause a wide range of respiratory symptoms. It may lead to severe illness, hospitalization, or death, especially in people with chronic medical conditions or a weakened immune system which increase their risk for severe illness.
- **Who Should Get It:** According to the latest CDC

guidance, all adults should stay current with COVID-19 vaccination.
- **Dosing Schedule:**
  - **Primary series:** Typically two doses of an mRNA vaccine, 3 – 4 weeks apart
  - **Boosters:** Given as needed based on updated strain recommendations and personal risk[15]

Men's Health Checklist: Ages 40 - 49

Bring this list to your next checkup. Use it to ask questions and ensure you're up to date on your preventive care.

Recommended Screenings

Screening	Completed	Notes
Blood Pressure	☐	
BMI and Metabolic Risk	☐	
Mental Health	☐	
HIV & STI	☐	
Lipid Panel (Cholesterol)	☐	
Diabetes	☐	
Colorectal Cancer (starts at 45)	☐	
Prostate Cancer	☐	
Vision Exam	☐	

Recommended Immunizations	Completed	Notes
Tdap (once if never received)	☐	Booster every 10 yrs.
Influenza (annually)	☐	Get every fall
COVID-19 (primary & booster(s))	☐	

Talk With Your Doctor About:

- Joint pain or stiffness
- Lack of mental focus, increased stress, or feelings of depression
- Sexual health, HIV and STI Prevention, and sexual performance
- Cancer screenings
- Sleep patterns or fatigue

CHAPTER 4
MEN IN THEIR 50S

Your 50s are a key decade for preventive health. During this stage of life, the risk of chronic conditions like heart disease, diabetes, cancer, and osteoporosis increases. Routine screenings and vaccinations are more important than ever for staying active, independent, and healthy into older adulthood.

RECOMMENDED SCREENINGS

1. Blood Pressure

Continue screening at least every 2 years, or annually if elevated.[1]

2. BMI and Weight Monitoring

Ongoing annual weight and BMI tracking is essential for managing obesity-related risks like type 2 diabetes, heart disease, and joint problems.[2]

3. Lipid Panel

Screen every 4 – 6 years for average-risk individuals, or more often if you have cardiovascular risk factors like diabetes, high blood pressure, or smoking history.[19]

4. Diabetes Screening

Continue screening every 3 years or more often for overweight men aged 40 – 70. Men with the following risk factors should be screened every 12 months to catch conversion to diabetes quickly and guide lifestyle changes and medication decisions.

1. History of gestational diabetes (in men, often a family history in a female partner may signal shared lifestyle risk)
2. Prediabetes (HbA1c 5.7–6.4%, fasting glucose 100 – 125 mg/dL)
3. Hypertension (≥140/90 mmHg or on therapy)
4. Low HDL (<35 mg/dL) or high triglycerides (>250 mg/dL)
5. History of heart disease or stroke
6. Family history – parent or sibling with diabetes

7. Black, Latino, Native American, Asian American, or Pacific Islander ethnicity
8. Sedentary lifestyle
9. Obesity or severe obesity[32]

Hemoglobin A1c and fasting glucose, both blood tests, are commonly used.[20]

5. Colorectal Cancer Screening

Colorectal cancer screening is essential and should continue if not already started at age 45. Screening options include:

- Colonoscopy every 10 years
- FIT annually
- CT colonography every 5 years, among others[21]

6. Prostate Cancer Screening

Continue shared decision-making with your doctor through age 69. Given high incidence and mortality rates, Black men should be screened every 1 – 2 years.[22, 32]

7. Lung Cancer Screening

Men aged 50 – 80 with a 20 pack-year smoking history who currently smoke or have quit within the last 15 years should be screened with low-dose CT annually.[24]

Understanding a 20-Pack-Year Smoking History

A pack-year is a way that doctors measures cigarette smoking over time. It multiples the number of packs of cigarettes that a person smokes each day by the number of years smoked.

How to Calculate Pack-Years:

Packs per Day	Years Smoked	Pack-Year Total
1 pack/day	20 years	20 pack-years
2 packs/day	10 years	20 pack-years
½ pack/day	40 years	20 pack-years

If your total is 20 pack-years or more, and you're between ages 50 and 80, you may qualify for annual lung cancer screening with a low-dose CT scan, especially if you currently smoke or quit smoking within the last 15 years. Discuss more with your doctor.

---

8. Osteoporosis Screening

Consider screening if you have risk factors like low body weight, smoking, steroid use, or family history of fractures. Men over 50 with a fracture may need a bone density scan (DEXA).[25]

9. Mental Health and Cognitive Function

Annual screening for depression and optional screening for mild cognitive impairment in those with concerns.[3]

10. Sexually Transmitted Infections (STIs)

Sexually active men should be screened for HIV at least once and every 3 – 6 months if you:

- have multiple sexual partners
- inject drugs or share drug equipment
- have condomless anal sex
- have a partner who is known to be living with HIV
- exchange sex for money, housing, or other resources
- have been diagnosed with a sexually transmitted infection (STI) in the past 6 months
- are using HIV pre-exposure prophylaxis (PrEP) – medication taken by mouth or as an injection to prevent HIV infection if you are exposed.[18]

Chlamydia, gonorrhea, and syphilis testing is also advised for those with multiple partners or other factors that increase the chances of getting an STI.[4]

☞ **For men who are having anal and/or oral sex:** If you are the receiving partner during anal sex (i.e., bottom or versatile) or give oral sex (i.e. you put your mouth on their genitals) to your sexual partners, you must ask your doctor to swab your anus and mouth to detect gonorrhea and/or chlamydia. A urine test will NOT detect gonorrhea or chlamydia in the anus or mouth.

RECOMMENDED IMMUNIZATIONS & DOSING SCHEDULES

By age 50, some new vaccines are added to your schedule, while others continue from earlier decades. Here's a breakdown by disease, including who needs it, when, how effective, and how long it lasts.

Shingles (Herpes Zoster) Vaccine

- **What It Protects Against:**
- Shingles—a painful rash caused by reactivation of the chickenpox virus. It can lead to postherpetic neuralgia, a long-lasting nerve pain.
- **Who Should Get It:**
    - Adults aged 50 and older, regardless of shingles or chickenpox history
- **Dosing Schedule:**
    - 2 doses, given 2 – 6 months apart
- **Effectiveness:**
    - Over 90% effective at preventing shingles and complications[26]
- **Duration:**
    - Protection lasts at least 7 years, possibly longer

Tetanus, Diphtheria, and Pertussis (Tdap) Vaccine

- **What It Protects Against:**
    - **Tetanus** – a serious bacterial infection that causes severe muscle stiffness, spasms, and can lead to death.
    - **Diphtheria** – a severe bacterial infection of the nose and throat that creates a thick, gray substance that covers the back of the throat, making breathing hard.
    - **Pertussis (whooping cough)** – a highly contagious bacterial infection that can cause violent coughing fits and is especially dangerous to infants.

- **Who Should Get It:** Adults who have never received Tdap.
- **Dosing Schedule:**
  - 1 dose of Tdap, then a Td or Tdap booster every 10 years[7].

☞ Most men completed the initial Tdap vaccine series during childhood, but you may be due for a booster.

- **Effectiveness & Duration:**
  - Tetanus/diphtheria: nearly 100% effective, lasts ~10 years
  - Pertussis: 69 – 85% effective, wanes after 1 – 2 years[12]

Influenza (Flu) Vaccine

- **What It Protects Against:**
  - The flu is a highly contagious respiratory illness that can cause fever, chills, fatigue, and body aches. It can also lead to serious complications, including pneumonia and hospitalization.
- **Who Should Get It:**
  - Annually, especially in fall
- **Effectiveness & Duration:**
  - 40 – 60% effective when matched well; lasts ~6 months[13]

COVID-19 Vaccine

- **What It Protects Against:**

- COVID-19 can cause a wide range of respiratory symptoms. It may lead to severe illness, hospitalization, or death, especially in people with chronic medical conditions or a weakened immune system which increase their risk for severe illness.
- **Who Should Get It:**
  - All adults, with boosters based on CDC guidance
- **Effectiveness & Duration:**
  - 90 – 95% effective after initial series; protection wanes after 4 – 6 months[15]

HPV Vaccine

- **Who Should Get It:**
  - Only if not vaccinated before age 27
  - Can be given to men up to age 45 if they have any of the following:
    - New or multiple sex partners
    - Men who have sex with men
    - Immunocompromised individuals, including those with HIV
    - Individuals who did not complete the vaccine series at a young age
    - History of STIs or inconsistent condom use
    - Partners with increased chance of having HPV (e.g., multiple partners or GBMSM)[6]

Pneumococcal Vaccine

- **What It Protects Against:**

- Pneumonia, sepsis, and meningitis caused by *Streptococcus pneumoniae*
- **Who Should Get It:**
  - Men aged 50+ with certain medical conditions (e.g., chronic heart, lung, liver disease, diabetes, smoking, immunocompromised)
  - Routine vaccination for all adults begins at age 65 (see next chapter)
- **Dosing Schedule:**
  - 1 dose of PCV20, or
  - PCV15 followed by PPSV23 1 year later (if using a sequential schedule)
- **Effectiveness:**
  - PCV20 and PCV15 both show > 85% effectiveness against invasive pneumococcal disease[27]
- **Duration:**
  - Long-lasting protection (several years); boosters may be required later

Men's Health Checklist: Ages 50 - 59

Bring this list to your next checkup. Use it to ask questions and ensure you're up to date on your preventive care.

Recommended Screenings

Screening	Completed	Notes
Blood Pressure	☐	Every 1 - 2 years
BMI and Weight	☐	
Mental Health	☐	
HIV & STI	☐	
Lipid Panel (Cholesterol)	☐	
Diabetes	☐	
Colorectal Cancer	☐	
Prostate Cancer	☐	
Vision and Hearing	☐	Every 1 - 2 years
Lung Cancer Screening	☐	20+ pack-year
Osteoporosis	☐	If risk factors

Recommended Immunizations

Immunization	Completed	Notes
Shingles	☐	Starts at age 50
Tdap (once if never received)	☐	Booster every 10 yrs.
Influenza (annually)	☐	Get every fall
COVID-19 (primary & booster(s))	☐	

Talk With Your Doctor About:

- Joint pain, strength, and flexibility
- Management of any chronic medical conditions
- Sexual health, HIV and STI Prevention, sexual performance, and testosterone levels
- Early signs of memory or mood changes

CHAPTER 5
MEN IN THEIR 60S

In your 60s, the focus shifts toward maintaining strength, independence, and mental sharpness. Chronic diseases may start to show symptoms, and subtle changes in balance, memory, or bone health can increase the risk of injury or decline. Preventive screenings and immunizations remain essential, and new vaccines—like those for pneumonia—are added to your care routine.

RECOMMENDED SCREENINGS

1. Blood Pressure

Continue at least every 1 – 2 years, or more often if elevated or on medication.[1]

2. BMI and Weight Monitoring

Continue annual weight, BMI, and waist circumference checks to track obesity-related risks.[2]

3. Lipid Panel

Recheck every 4 – 6 years, or more frequently if you have heart disease or diabetes.[19]

4. Diabetes Screening

Screening should continue every 3 years for people without risk factors for diabetes.[20] Men with the following risk factors should be screened every 12 months to catch conversion to diabetes quickly and guide lifestyle changes and medication decisions.

1. History of gestational diabetes (in men, often a family history in a female partner may signal shared lifestyle risk)
2. Prediabetes (HbA1c 5.7 – 6.4%, fasting glucose 100 – 125 mg/dL)
3. Hypertension (≥140/90 mmHg or on therapy)
4. Low HDL (<35 mg/dL) or high triglycerides (>250 mg/dL)
5. History of heart disease or stroke
6. Family history – parent or sibling with diabetes
7. Black, Latino, Native American, Asian American, or Pacific Islander ethnicity
8. Sedentary lifestyle

9. Obesity or severe obesity[32]

Hemoglobin A1c and fasting glucose, both blood tests, are commonly used.[20]

5. Colorectal Cancer Screening

- Continue until at least age 75 using:
- Colonoscopy (every 10 years)
- FIT test (annually)
- CT colonography (every 5 years), etc.[21]

6. Prostate Cancer Screening

Continue shared decision-making with your doctor through age 69. Given high incidence and mortality rates, Black men should be screened every 1 – 2 years. [22, 32]

7. Lung Cancer Screening

Continue annual low-dose CT scans if you meet all of the following:

- Ages 50 – 80
- 20 pack-year smoking history
- Currently smoke or quit within the past 15 years[24]

Understanding a 20-Pack-Year Smoking History

A pack-year is a way that doctors measures cigarette smoking over time. It multiplies the number of packs of cigarettes that a person smokes each day by the number of years smoked.

How to Calculate Pack-Years:

Packs per Day	Years Smoked	Pack-Year Total
1 pack/day	20 years	20 pack-years
2 packs/day	10 years	20 pack-years
½ pack/day	40 years	20 pack-years

If your total is 20 pack-years or more, and you're between ages 50 and 80, you may qualify for annual lung cancer screening with a low-dose CT scan, especially if you currently smoke or quit smoking within the last 15 years. Discuss more with your doctor.

8. Osteoporosis Screening

Men over age 65 or younger with risk factors (e.g., low body weight, prior fractures, steroid use) should be screened with a DEXA scan.[25]

9. Vision and Hearing

- Eye exams every 1 – 2 years
- Hearing test every 1 – 3 years, or sooner if there are signs of hearing loss[23]

10. Fall Risk and Balance Screening

Annual screening using simple tests (e.g., Timed Up and Go) can help prevent serious injuries from falls.[28]

11. Mental Health and Cognitive Screening

Continue depression screening as older men may underreport symptoms. Consider a brief memory screening if you or your family notice changes in attention, language, or recall.[3,29]

12. Sexually Transmitted Infections (STIs)

Sexually active men should be screened for HIV at least once and every 3 – 6 months if you:

- have multiple sexual partners
- inject drugs or share drug equipment
- have condomless anal sex
- have a partner who is known to be living with HIV
- exchange sex for money, housing, or other resources
- have been diagnosed with a sexually transmitted infection (STI) in the past 6 months
- are using HIV pre-exposure prophylaxis (PrEP) – medication taken by mouth or as an injection to prevent HIV infection if you are exposed.[18]

Chlamydia, gonorrhea, and syphilis testing is also advised for those with multiple partners or other factors that increase the chances of getting and STI.[4]

☞ **For men who are having anal and/or oral sex:** If you are the receiving partner during anal sex (i.e., bottom or versatile) or give oral sex (i.e. you put your mouth on their genitals) to your sexual partners, you must ask your doctor to swab your anus and mouth to detect gonorrhea and/or chlamydia. A urine test will NOT detect gonorrhea or chlamydia in the anus or mouth.

RECOMMENDED IMMUNIZATIONS & DOSING SCHEDULES

The immune system begins to decline with age, increasing the risk of serious illness from common infections. The following vaccines are vital in one's 60s and beyond.

Shingles (Herpes Zoster) Vaccine

- **What It Protects Against:**
- Shingles—a painful rash caused by reactivation of the chickenpox virus. It can lead to postherpetic neuralgia, a long-lasting nerve pain.
- **Who Should Get It:**
    - All adults age 50 and older
- **Dosing Schedule:**
    - 2 doses, 2 – 6 months apart
- **Effectiveness:**
    - Over 90% effective at preventing shingles and postherpetic neuralgia[26]
- **Duration:**
    - Lasts at least 7 years

Pneumococcal Vaccine (PCV20 or PCV15 + PPSV23)

- **What It Protects Against:**

- Pneumonia, sepsis, and meningitis caused by the bacteria *Streptococcus pneumoniae*
- **Who Should Get It:**
  - All adults age 65+
  - Adults aged 19 – 64 with risk factors (e.g., smoking, heart/lung disease, diabetes, immunocompromised)[27]
- **Dosing Schedule:**
  - Option 1: 1 dose of PCV20
  - Option 2: 1 dose of PCV15, then 1 dose of PPSV23 1 year later
- **Effectiveness:**
  - Over 85% effective against invasive pneumococcal disease
- **Duration:**
  - Several years; boosters not routinely required if PCV20 is used

Tetanus, Diphtheria, and Pertussis (Tdap) Vaccine

- **What It Protects Against:**
  - **Tetanus** – a serious bacterial infection that causes severe muscle stiffness, spasms, and can lead to death.
  - **Diphtheria** – a severe bacterial infection of the nose and throat that creates a thick, gray substance that covers the back of the throat, making breathing hard.
  - **Pertussis (whooping cough)** – a highly contagious

bacterial infection that can cause violent coughing fits and is especially dangerous to infants.
- **Who Should Get It:** Adults who have never received the Tdap vaccine.
- **Dosing Schedule:**
  - 1 dose of Tdap, then a booster every 10 years[7].

☞ Most men completed the initial Tdap vaccine series during childhood, but you may be due for a booster.

- **Effectiveness & Duration:**
  - **Tetanus/diphtheria:** nearly 100% effective; 10-year protection
  - **Pertussis:** 69 – 85% effective; wanes after 1 – 2 years[12]

Influenza (Flu) Vaccine

- **What It Protects Against:**
  - The flu is a highly contagious respiratory illness that can cause fever, chills, fatigue, and body aches. It can also lead to serious complications, including pneumonia and hospitalization.
- **Who Should Get It:**
  - All adults annually, high-dose or adjuvanted vaccine recommended for adults ≥ 65
- **Dosing Schedule:**
  - 1 dose every year, ideally before flu season
- **Effectiveness:**
  - Reduces serious illness, hospitalizations, and death

- High-dose flu vaccine may be 24% more effective in older adults[31]
- **Duration:**
  - Approximately 6 months

COVID-19 Vaccine

- **What It Protects Against:**
  - COVID-19 can cause a wide range of respiratory symptoms. It may lead to severe illness, hospitalization, or death, especially in people with chronic medical conditions or a weakened immune system which increase their risk for severe illness.
- **Who Should Get It:**
  - All adults, especially older adults and those with chronic conditions
- **Dosing Schedule:**
  - Follow current CDC guidance (typically boosters every 6 – 12 months)
- **Effectiveness:**
  - Initial series: 90 – 95% effective
  - Boosters maintain protection as it declines with time[15]
- **Duration:**
  - 4 – 6 months; booster needed to sustain immunity

Men's Health Checklist: Ages 60 - 69

Bring this list to your next checkup. Use it to ask questions and ensure you're up to date on your preventive care.

Recommended Screenings

Screening	Completed	Notes
Blood Pressure	☐	Every 1 - 2 years
Weight and Muscle Loss	☐	
Cognitive and Mental Health	☐	
HIV & STI	☐	
Lipid Panel (Cholesterol)	☐	
Diabetes	☐	
Colorectal Cancer	☐	
Prostate Cancer	☐	
Vision and Hearing	☐	Every 1 - 2 years
Lung Cancer Screening	☐	20+ pack-year
Osteoporosis and Risk of Falls	☐	If risk factors

Recommended Immunizations

Recommended Immunizations	Completed	Notes
Pneumococcal	☐	
Shingles	☐	Starts at age 50
Tdap (once if never received)	☐	Booster every 10 yrs.
Influenza (annually)	☐	Get every fall
COVID-19 (primary & booster(s))	☐	

Talk With Your Doctor About:

- Management of any chronic medical conditions
- Sexual health, HIV/STI Prevention, sexual performance, and testosterone levels
- Early signs of memory or mood changes
- Preventing falls and maintaining ability to walk well
- Home safety and independence

CHAPTER 6
MEN 70 AND OLDER

As men enter their 70s and beyond, health priorities shift toward preserving independence, mobility, mental sharpness, and social engagement. Many age-related conditions, like falls, frailty, cognitive decline, and vision or hearing loss, become more common. Screening and prevention efforts should be based on your overall health and the number of years that you are expected to live. Maintaining a close relationship with your doctor is key.

RECOMMENDED SCREENINGS

1. Blood Pressure

Continue monitoring at least annually, especially if on blood pressure medication.[1]

2. BMI, Nutrition, and Muscle Loss

Track weight, BMI, and muscle mass to prevent loss of muscle tissue and becoming weak. Unintentional weight loss is a red flag for underlying issues. Talk to your doctor if you notice changes in your weight.[2]

3. Diabetes and Lipid Screening

Continue if at risk or previously diagnosed. Ask your doctor about your current doses of medication to determine if they can be decreased, particularly if intensive control of diabetes is causing harm, such as causing episodes of low blood sugar and feeling faint, which increases the risk for falls.[20]

4. Colorectal Cancer Screening

Stop routine screening around age 75 or when life expectancy is <10 years unless prior polyps or high risk.[21]

5. Prostate Cancer Screening

Routine PSA screening is not recommended after age 70 per USPSTF due to limited benefit[22]—but some guidelines allow shared decision-making in healthy older men. According to the American Urological Association and other expert groups, continued screening may be considered in the following men:

> **Excellent functional status and life expectancy ≥10 years**
> - For example, active 70 – 75-year-olds with no major health problems

A strong family history of prostate cancer
- Especially if a first-degree relative, such as your brother or father, was diagnosed before age 60

Black men
- Who face higher rates of prostate cancer and more aggressive disease[32]

Men with a personal history of elevated PSA or abnormal findings

6. Lung Cancer Screening

Continue annual low-dose CT scans through age 80 if you have a 20 pack-year history and meet criteria.[24]

Understanding a 20-Pack-Year Smoking History

A pack-year is a way that doctors measures cigarette smoking over time. It multiples the number of packs of cigarettes that a person smokes each day by the number of years smoked.

How to Calculate Pack-Years:

Packs per Day	Years Smoked	Pack-Year Total
1 pack/day	20 years	20 pack-years
2 packs/day	10 years	20 pack-years
½ pack/day	40 years	20 pack-years

If your total is 20 pack-years or more, and you're between ages 50 and 80, you may qualify for annual lung cancer screening with a low-dose CT scan, especially if you currently smoke or quit smoking within the last 15 years. Discuss more with your doctor.

---

7. Osteoporosis and Fall Risk

Get screened for osteoporosis with a DEXA scan if not done earlier. Ask your doctor for tests to assess your risk for falls.[25,28]

8. Vision and Hearing

Eye exam every 1 – 2 years
Hearing check annually, or sooner with hearing changes[23]

9. Cognitive and Mental Health Screening

Consider screening for mild cognitive impairment if symptoms are present
Continue depression screening as older men may underreport symptoms[3,29]

10. Sexually Transmitted Infections (STIs)

Sexually active men should be screened for HIV at least once and every 3 – 6 months if you:

- have multiple sexual partners
- inject drugs or share drug equipment
- have condomless anal sex
- have a partner who is known to be living with HIV
- exchange sex for money, housing, or other resources
- have been diagnosed with a sexually transmitted infection (STI) in the past 6 months
- are using HIV pre-exposure prophylaxis (PrEP) – medication taken by mouth or as an injection to prevent HIV infection if you are exposed.[18]

Chlamydia, gonorrhea, and syphilis testing is also advised for those with multiple partners or other factors that increase the chances of getting an STI.[4]

☞ **For men who are having anal and/or oral sex:** If you are the receiving partner during anal sex (i.e., bottom or versatile) or give oral sex (i.e. you put your mouth on their genitals) to your sexual partners, you must ask your doctor to swab your anus and mouth to detect gonorrhea and/or chlamydia. A urine test will NOT detect gonorrhea or chlamydia in the anus or mouth.

RECOMMENDED IMMUNIZATIONS & DOSING SCHEDULES

Vaccinations remain essential in this age group to prevent hospitalizations, disability, and death—especially from respiratory or vaccine-preventable illnesses.

1. Shingles (Herpes Zoster) Vaccine

- **What It Protects Against:**
- Shingles—a painful rash caused by reactivation of the chickenpox virus. It can lead to postherpetic neuralgia, a long-lasting nerve pain.
- **Who Should Get It:**
    - All adults 50+, even if they had shingles before or received Zostavax
- **Dosing Schedule:**
    - 2 doses of Shingrix, 2 – 6 months apart
- **Effectiveness:**

- Over 90% effective in preventing shingles and long-term nerve pain[26]
- **Duration:**
  - Protection lasts at least 7 years

2. Pneumococcal Vaccine (PCV20 or PCV15 + PPSV23)

- **What It Protects Against:**
- Pneumonia, sepsis, and meningitis caused by *Streptococcus pneumoniae*
- **Who Should Get It:**
  - All adults age 65+
- **Dosing Options:**
  - PCV20: Single dose
  - PCV15 + PPSV23: PCV15 followed by PPSV23 at least 1 year later[27]
- **Effectiveness:**
  - 85% against invasive pneumococcal disease (i.e., severe pneumonia)
- **Duration:**
  - Lasts several years

3. Tetanus, Diphtheria, and Pertussis (Tdap) Vaccine

- **What It Protects Against:**
  - **Tetanus** – a serious bacterial infection that causes severe muscle stiffness, spasms, and can lead to death.
  - **Diphtheria** – a severe bacterial infection of the nose and throat that creates a thick, gray substance that

covers the back of the throat, making breathing hard.
  - **Pertussis (whooping cough)** – a highly contagious bacterial infection that can cause violent coughing fits and is especially dangerous to infants.
- **Who Should Get It:** Adults who have never received the Tdap vaccine.
- **Dosing Schedule:**
  - 1 dose of Tdap, then a booster every 10 years[7].

☞ Most men completed the initial Tdap vaccine series during childhood, but you may be due for a booster.

- **Effectiveness & Duration:**
  - Tetanus/diphtheria: nearly 100%, 10-year duration
  - Pertussis: 69 – 85% effective, wanes after 1 – 2 years[12]

4. Influenza Vaccine (High-Dose or Adjuvanted)

- **What It Protects Against:**
  - The flu is a highly contagious respiratory illness that can cause fever, chills, fatigue, and body aches. It can also lead to serious complications, including pneumonia and hospitalization.
- **Who Should Get It:**
  - All adults annually; high-dose or adjuvanted vaccine preferred in people ages 65 or older
- **Effectiveness:**
  - High-dose flu vaccine is more effective in older adults[30]

- **Duration:**
  - Lasts approximately 6 months

5. **COVID-19 Vaccine**

- **What It Protects Against:**
  - COVID-19 can cause a wide range of respiratory symptoms. It may lead to severe illness, hospitalization, or death, especially in people with chronic medical conditions or a weakened immune system which increase their risk for severe illness.
- **Who Should Get It:**
  - All older adults, especially those with chronic illness or living in group settings
- **Dosing Schedule:**
  - Follow current CDC guidance, typically a booster every 6 – 12 months
- **Effectiveness:**
  - 90 – 95% after initial series; boosters restore declining immunity[15]
- **Duration:**
  - Approximately 4 – 6 months

Men's Health Checklist: Ages 70+

Bring this list to your next checkup. Use it to ask questions and ensure you're up to date on your preventive care.

Recommended Screenings

Screening	Completed	Notes
Blood Pressure	☐	Every 1 - 2 years
BMI and Nutrition	☐	
Cognitive and Mental Health	☐	
HIV & STI	☐	
Lipid Panel (Cholesterol)	☐	Talk with your doctor.
Diabetes	☐	Talk with your doctor.
Colorectal Cancer	☐	Stop after 75 if low risk
Prostate Cancer	☐	Talk with your doctor.
Vision and Hearing	☐	Every 1 - 2 years
Lung Cancer Screening	☐	Continue to age 80
Osteoporosis and Risk of Falls	☐	

Recommended Immunizations

Immunization	Completed	Notes
Pneumococcal	☐	
Shingles	☐	Starts at age 50
Tdap (once if never received)	☐	Booster every 10 yrs.
Influenza (annually)	☐	Get every fall
COVID-19 (primary & booster(s))	☐	

Talk With Your Doctor About:

- Staying independent and active
- Memory, cognition, and safety concerns
- Need for certain medications given risk of overmedication with age
- Social connection and caregiver support
- End-of-life preferences and planning

CHAPTER 7
SPECIAL POPULATIONS

Health guidelines often follow a "one-size-fits-all" model, but many men live with unique health challenges or barriers that require personalized care. This chapter focuses on special populations of men who may need modified screenings, earlier interventions, or additional vaccines to achieve equitable health outcomes.

GAY, BI, AND OTHER MEN WHO HAVE SEX WITH MEN (GBMSM)

GBMSM experience higher rates of HIV, STIs, HPV-related cancers, and often experience mental health disparities due to stigma and discrimination.

Screening Recommendations:

- HIV testing every 3 – 6 months if sexually active with new or multiple partners or using PrEP[18]
- Mental health and substance use screening at regular checkups
- Annual STI testing: chlamydia, gonorrhea, syphilis, and hepatitis B and C[4]

☞ For men who are having anal and/or oral sex: If you are the receiving partner during anal sex (i.e., bottom or versatile) or give oral sex (i.e. you put your mouth on their genitals) to your sexual partners, you must ask your doctor to swab your anus and mouth to detect gonorrhea and/or chlamydia. A urine test will NOT detect gonorrhea or chlamydia in the anus or mouth.

- Anal cancer screening for GBMSM living with HIV or with other risk factors, such as:
    - GBMSM with persistent or high-risk HPV infection, with types of HPV such as 16 and 18, which can cause cancer
    - History of genital warts
    - History of cervical or vulvar cancer in female partners
    - People with weakened immune systems (not only people living with HIV, but also those with cancer on chemotherapy or others with autoimmune diseases like Lupus on steroids or other medications that weaken the immune system).
    - Current or past history of smoking[37,38]

SPECIAL POPULATIONS

☞ Currently, there are not clear guidelines for anal cancer screening for people who are not living with HIV. If you engage in anal insertive sex or are the bottom partner, talk with your doctor about anal cancer screening. For People living with HIV, see the *"People Living with HIV"* section below for more details on anal cancer screening recommendations and the tests that are conducted for screening.

Doxycycline for STI Prevention:

A new option called doxycycline post-exposure prophylaxis (or DoxyPEP) can help reduce your chances of getting syphilis, gonorrhea, and chlamydia from condomless sex. DoxyPEP involves taking a 200 mg dose of the antibiotic doxycycline within 72 hours after sex to prevent infection. The Centers for Disease Control and Prevention (CDC) recommends DoxyPEP for gay, bisexual, and other men who have sex with men who had an STI like syphilis, gonorrhea, or chlamydia in the past year.[50]

Research shows DoxyPEP decreases the chance of getting syphilis by 70% to 80%, and it lowers the risk of chlamydia by about 65% to 90%.[51,52] It may also help reduce gonorrhea, although the results are mixed. In some studies, DoxyPEP lowered the risk of gonorrhea by about 50%, while in others, it only lowered it by 20%. Overall, this option can be very effective in preventing STIs. I encourage you to discuss further with your doctor if you think it could be a great fit for you.[53]

Immunizations:

- HPV vaccine through age 26; consider through age 45 based on risk. *See Chapters 1, 2, or 3, based on your age.*[6]
- Hepatitis A and B vaccines if not already immune[34]
- Meningococcal MenACWY vaccine during community outbreaks[14]

VETERANS

Military service can expose men to unique physical and psychological risks, including trauma, chronic pain, and environmental exposures.

Focus Areas:

- Mental health screening for PTSD, depression, and suicide risk
- Hepatitis C screening (especially if born between 1945 and 1965 or exposed during service)[35]
- Hearing and vision assessments due to service-related damage
- Musculoskeletal evaluations for chronic pain, arthritis, or injury
- Sleep and substance use evaluations

MEN WITH CHRONIC CONDITIONS

Chronic illnesses, like diabetes, HIV, cardiovascular disease, or cancer, often require earlier, more frequent, or expanded screenings.

Modified Screening and Immunization Considerations:

- Annual eye exams and foot checks for men with diabetes[36]
- Kidney function screening in diabetes
- Earlier pneumococcal vaccination if heart, lung, liver disease, or diabetes is present[27]
- More frequent lipid, Hemoglobin A1c, and liver function testing

MEN WITH DISABILITIES

Men with cognitive, physical, or developmental disabilities often receive fewer screenings and may face caregiver-related barriers.

Areas of Focus:

- Accessible facilities and communication support
- Routine cancer screenings
- Abuse and neglect screening in institutional or dependent settings
- Coordination with caregivers and support systems

PEOPLE LIVING WITH HIV

Living with HIV doesn't mean putting your health on pause. It means being even more intentional about your preventive care. Regular checkups, screenings, and open conversations with your doctor can help you stay strong, stay ahead of health issues, and keep living well. As a person living with HIV, starting on treatment and staying on it is key. Your goal is to become undetectable. Being *undetectable* means there's so little virus in your blood that standard tests can't measure it, and it also means you can't pass HIV to your sexual partners. This is called U=U, or Undetectable = Untransmittable.[39] Being undetectable also helps preserve your white blood cells, helping you maintain a healthy immune system to fight infections.

One key area of preventive care is anal cancer screening, especially for gay, bi, and other men who have sex with men (GBMSM), people living with HIV, and those with a history of genital warts. People living with HIV are at higher risk for anal cancer due to long-term HPV (human papillomavirus) infection. Screening helps catch early changes before they become cancer.[37,41]

For people living with HIV, regardless of age, every year, an assessment of any anal symptoms such as unexplained itching, anal bleeding, or pain, as well as presence of any sores in the anus is recommended. Completion of a digital anal rectal exam (DARE) once a year is also recommended.[49] This exam involves a gloved finger inserted into the anus to gently check the anal canal for any lumps or unusual areas.

For men living with HIV who have sex with other men:

- If you are under the age of 35 and have any of the anal symptoms mentioned above, having a standard anoscopy is recommended.

- If you are over the age of 35 and have any of the anal symptoms mentioned above, skipping the standard anoscopy and going directly to the high-resolution anoscopy (HRA), which is a more specialized test, is recommended.

For men living with HIV who do not have sex with other men:

- If you are under the age of 45 and have any of the anal symptoms mentioned above, having a standard anoscopy is recommended.
- If you are over the age of 45 and have any of the anal symptoms mentioned above, skipping the standard anoscopy and going directly to the high-resolution anoscopy (HRA), which is a more specialized test, is recommended.[49]

Below are a few helpful definitions:

- A standard anoscopy, sometimes referred to as an anal Pap smear, is a vital test that checks for early signs of cancer in the anus. It involves a doctor or nurse inserting a thin, hollow instrument called an anoscope into the anus to examine the internal structures of the anus and lower rectum. They then gently insert a small swab, similar to a Q-tip), through the hollow tube to collect a sample of the cells inside the anus. These cells are then examined under a microscope to detect unusual or harmful changes.

- A high-resolution anoscopy is a test that uses a special microscope to examine your anal canal closely. It is quick and if they see anything that looks unusual, they will take a small sample of tissue, which is called a biopsy, to examine more closely in a lab.[41]

In addition to anal cancer screening, other screenings and vaccines are vital for people living with HIV:

- Hepatitis A, B, and C screening: Everyone living with HIV should be tested at least once. If you're not already immune, you should get vaccinated for hepatitis A and B.[42]
- Tuberculosis (TB) screening: A TB test is recommended at diagnosis. If you're at ongoing risk, it may be repeated each year.[43]
- Sexually transmitted infections (STIs): Screen for syphilis, gonorrhea, and chlamydia at least once a year, or more often if you have new or multiple partners.[44]
- Lung cancer screening: If you're age 50 to 80, have a history of heavy smoking, and currently smoke or quit within the past 15 years, a low-dose CT scan may be recommended.[24]

Let's talk about vaccines. Staying up to date with your shots is a huge part of staying well. For people living with HIV, the following are often recommended:

- HPV vaccine (up to age 45) to reduce the risk of HPV-related cancers[6]

SPECIAL POPULATIONS

- Meningococcal vaccine (MenACWY) - initial dose and a booster every 5 years[34]
- Hepatitis A and B vaccines (if not already immune)[49]
- Pneumococcal vaccine - either PCV20 alone or PCV15 followed by PPSV23[50]
- Mpox (monkeypox) vaccine - recommended for those at higher risk, including people with HIV who have multiple sex partners[46]
- COVID-19 vaccines and boosters[47]
- Flu shot every year[48]

☞ Some live vaccines may be unsafe if your CD4 count, the number of a type of white blood cells, is under 200. Your doctor can help decide what's best based on your immune status.

Bottom line: Living with HIV is manageable, and with the proper care, you can thrive and live a long, healthy life. Ask questions, speak up for your needs, and work with doctors who see and support the whole you.

APPENDIX

HOW TO DO A TESTICULAR SELF-EXAM

When to Do It:

- Once a month
- The best time is during or right after a warm shower or bath (your skin is relaxed)

Instructions:

Step 1: Get ready

Stand in front of a mirror. Look for any swelling or changes in the size or shape of your testicles.

Step 2: Use both hands

Hold one testicle at a time. Use your thumb and fingers to roll it around gently.

Step 3: Feel for any changes

You're checking for:

- Lumps (even small ones)
- Hard spots
- Pain or tenderness

A soft tube (called the epididymis) is normal behind each testicle. That's not a lump!

Step 4: Repeat on the other side

Check both testicles the same way.

Step 5: If something feels different

Don't panic—but don't wait. Tell a parent, guardian, or doctor right away.

GLOSSARY OF ACRONYMS & DEFINITIONS

ADA – *American Diabetes Association*

An organization that publishes guidelines for managing and preventing diabetes.

AUA – *American Urological Association*

A professional group focused on urologic health, including prostate care.

BMI – *Body Mass Index*

A measure of body fat based on your height and weight.

BP – *Blood Pressure*

The force of your blood pushing against the walls of your arteries.

CDC – *Centers for Disease Control and Prevention*

GLOSSARY OF ACRONYMS & DEFINITIONS

A U.S. agency that provides public health guidance and disease prevention info.

COVID-19 – *Coronavirus Disease 2019*

A viral illness that can cause fever, cough, and breathing problems.

CVD – *Cardiovascular Disease*

Diseases related to the heart and blood vessels.

DARE – *Digital anal rectal exam*

Examination in which a doctor inserts a finger gently inside the anal canal to check for any lumps or unusual areas.

DEXA – *Dual-Energy X-ray Absorptiometry*

A special scan is used to measure bone strength and check for osteoporosis.

FIT – *Fecal Immunochemical Test*

A stool test for hidden blood is used to screen for colon cancer.

HbA1c – *Hemoglobin A1c*

A blood test that shows your average blood sugar levels over the past 2–3 months.

HIV – *Human Immunodeficiency Virus*

A virus that weakens the immune system and can lead to AIDS if untreated.

HPV – *Human Papillomavirus*

GLOSSARY OF ACRONYMS & DEFINITIONS

HPV is a common virus that can cause genital warts and certain types of cancer.

HRA – *High-Resolution Anoscopy*

A close-up exam of the anal area to check for signs of cancer or pre-cancer.

LGBTQ+ – *Lesbian, Gay, Bisexual, Transgender, Queer/Questioning, and others*

A term for people with diverse sexual orientations and gender identities.

GBMSM – *Gay, Bi, and Other Men Who Have Sex with Men*

A medical term used to describe gay men, bisexual men, or other men who engage in sexual activity with other men.

OGTT – *Oral Glucose Tolerance Test*

A test that checks how your body handles sugar, used to screen for diabetes.

PCV – *Pneumococcal Conjugate Vaccine*

A vaccine that protects against a type of bacteria that can cause pneumonia.

PPSV – *Pneumococcal Polysaccharide Vaccine*

Another form of pneumonia vaccine, used in older adults and high-risk people.

PSA – *Prostate-Specific Antigen*

A protein made by the prostate; high levels can be a sign of prostate cancer.

PTSD – *Post-Traumatic Stress Disorder*

A mental health condition caused by very stressful or scary events.

STI – *Sexually Transmitted Infection*

Infections passed from person to person through sexual contact.

TBI – *Traumatic Brain Injury*

Damage to the brain from a blow, fall, or other head injury—often seen in veterans.

Td – *Tetanus and Diphtheria Vaccine*

A booster shot for adults to safeguard against tetanus and diphtheria.

Tdap – *Tetanus, Diphtheria, and Pertussis Vaccine*

Protects against three diseases, including whooping cough.

USPSTF – *U.S. Preventive Services Task Force*

A group that reviews research and makes screening recommendations.

THANK YOU

FOUND THIS GUIDE HELPFUL?
SPREAD THE WORD!

Your journey to better health and stronger self-advocacy starts now, and I'm honored that *The Men's Preventive Health Guide* is part of it.

If you found this guide helpful, I have two requests:

1. Please tell other men about it. We must get this book into the hands of as many men as possible to have the fullest impact.
2. Please leave a short review on the website where you purchased the book. Your feedback will help more men (and the people who love them) discover this resource and make empowered choices about their health.

Your voice matters—and your actions can truly make a difference.

BIBLIOGRAPHY

1. U.S. Preventive Services Task Force. **Final Recommendation Statement: High Blood Pressure in Adults: Screening**. 2021. Available at: https://www.uspreventiveservicestaskforce.org
2. Centers for Disease Control and Prevention (CDC). **About Adult BMI**. Updated March 1, 2022. Available at: https://www.cdc.gov/healthyweight/assessing/bmi/adult_bmi/index.html
3. Siu AL; U.S. Preventive Services Task Force. **Screening for Depression in Adults: U.S. Preventive Services Task Force Recommendation Statement**. *JAMA*. 2016;315(4):380-387.
4. Centers for Disease Control and Prevention (CDC). **Sexually Transmitted Infections Treatment Guidelines, 2021**. *MMWR Recomm Rep*. 2021;70(4):1–187.
5. U.S. Preventive Services Task Force. **Testicular Cancer: Screening**. 2011. Available at: https://www.uspreventiveservicestaskforce.org
6. Meites E, Szilagyi PG, Chesson HW, et al. **Human Papillomavirus Vaccination for Adults: Updated Recommendations of the Advisory Committee on Immunization Practices**. *MMWR Morb Mortal Wkly Rep*. 2019;68(32):698–702.
7. CDC. **Tdap (Tetanus, Diphtheria, Pertussis) Vaccine Recommendations**. Updated 2023. Available at: https://www.cdc.gov/vaccines/vpd/tdap/recs.html
8. CDC. **Influenza (Flu) Vaccine: Who Should Get Vaccinated**. Available at: https://www.cdc.gov/flu/prevent/vaccinations.htm
9. CDC. **Meningococcal Vaccination: What Everyone Should Know**. Updated October 16, 2023. Available at: https://www.cdc.gov/vaccines/vpd/mening/public/index.html
10. CDC. **Stay Up to Date with COVID-19 Vaccines**. Updated 2024. Available at: https://www.cdc.gov/coronavirus/2019-ncov/vaccines/stay-up-to-date.html
11. Garland SM, Kjaer SK, Muñoz N, et al. **Impact and Effectiveness of the Quadrivalent Human Papillomavirus Vaccine: A Systematic**

BIBLIOGRAPHY

Review of 10 Years of Real-world Experience. *Clin Infect Dis.* 2016;63(4):519–527.

12. Acosta AM, DeBolt C, Tasslimi A, et al. **Tetanus, Diphtheria, and Acellular Pertussis Vaccines: Use in Adults and Adolescents.** *MMWR Morb Mortal Wkly Rep.* 2015;64(31):831–835.

13. CDC. **Vaccine Effectiveness: How Well Do Flu Vaccines Work?** Updated December 7, 2023. Available at: https://www.cdc.gov/flu/vaccines-work/vaccineeffect.htm

14. MacNeil JR, Rubin L, Folaranmi T, et al. **Use of Serogroup B Meningococcal Vaccines in Adolescents and Young Adults: Recommendations of the Advisory Committee on Immunization Practices (ACIP), 2015.** *MMWR Morb Mortal Wkly Rep.* 2015;64(41):1171–1176.

15. Polack FP, Thomas SJ, Kitchin N, et al. **Safety and Efficacy of the BNT162b2 mRNA COVID-19 Vaccine.** *N Engl J Med.* 2020;383(27):2603–2615.

16. Basta NE, Shapiro ED. **Meningococcal Vaccines and Vaccine Strategies.** *Pediatrics.* 2019;144(1):e20182584.

17. Ostergaard L, Vesikari T, Absalon J, et al. **A Bivalent Meningococcal B Vaccine in Adolescents and Young Adults.** *N Engl J Med.* 2017;377(23):2349–2362.

18. CDC. **HIV Testing Overview: Who Should Get Tested and When.** Updated August 2023. Available at: https://www.cdc.gov/hiv/basics/testing.html

19. Stone NJ, Robinson JG, Lichtenstein AH, et al. **2013 ACC/AHA Guideline on the Treatment of Blood Cholesterol to Reduce Atherosclerotic Cardiovascular Risk in Adults**: A Report of the American College of Cardiology/American Heart Association Task Force on Practice Guidelines. *Circulation.* 2014;129(25 Suppl 2):S1–S45. doi:10.1161/01.cir.0000437738.63853.7a

20. US Preventive Services Task Force (USPSTF); Davidson KW, Barry MJ, Mangione CM, et al. **Screening for Prediabetes and Type 2 Diabetes: US Preventive Services Task Force Recommendation Statement.** *JAMA.* 2021;326(8):736–743. doi:10.1001/jama.2021.12531

21. US Preventive Services Task Force (USPSTF); Davidson KW, Barry MJ, Mangione CM, et al. **Screening for Colorectal Cancer: US**

Preventive Services Task Force Recommendation Statement. *JAMA*. 2021;325(19):1965–1977. doi:10.1001/jama.2021.6238

22. US Preventive Services Task Force (USPSTF); Grossman DC, Curry SJ, Owens DK, et al. **Screening for Prostate Cancer: US Preventive Services Task Force Recommendation Statement**. *JAMA*. 2018;319(18):1901–1913. doi:10.1001/jama.2018.3710

23. American Academy of Ophthalmology. **Eye Health Guidelines for Adults Over 40**. Updated October 2022. Available at: https://www.aao.org/eye-health/tips-prevention/adult-eye-exams

24. US Preventive Services Task Force (USPSTF); Krist AH, Davidson KW, Mangione CM, et al. **Screening for Lung Cancer: US Preventive Services Task Force Recommendation Statement**. *JAMA*. 2021;325(10):962–970. doi:10.1001/jama.2021.1117

25. Qaseem A, Forciea MA, McLean RM, Denberg TD; Clinical Guidelines Committee of the American College of Physicians. **Treatment of Low Bone Density or Osteoporosis to Prevent Fractures in Men and Women: A Clinical Practice Guideline Update From the American College of Physicians**. *Ann Intern Med*. 2017;166(11):818–839. doi:10.7326/M15-1361

26. Cunningham AL, Lal H, Kovac M, et al. **Efficacy of the Herpes Zoster Subunit Vaccine in Adults 50 Years of Age or Older**. *N Engl J Med*. 2016;375(11):1019–1032. doi:10.1056/NEJMoa1608653

27. CDC. **Pneumococcal Vaccination: Summary of Who and When to Vaccinate**. Updated September 14, 2023. Available at: https://www.cdc.gov/vaccines/vpd/pneumo/hcp/who-when-to-vaccinate.html

28. Panel on Prevention of Falls in Older Persons, American Geriatrics Society and British Geriatrics Society. **Summary of the Updated American Geriatrics Society/British Geriatrics Society Clinical Practice Guideline for Prevention of Falls in Older Persons**. *J Am Geriatr Soc*. 2011;59(1):148–157. doi:10.1111/j.1532-5415.2010.03234.x

29. Moyer VA; U.S. Preventive Services Task Force. **Screening for Cognitive Impairment in Older Adults: U.S. Preventive Services Task Force Recommendation Statement**. *Ann Intern Med*. 2014;160(11):791–797. doi:10.7326/M14-0496

30. Diaz Granados CA, Dunning AJ, Kimmel M, et al. **Efficacy of High-Dose versus Standard-Dose Influenza Vaccine in Older Adults**. *N*

Engl J Med. 2014;371(7):635–645. doi:10.1056/NEJMoa1315727

31. Carlsson SV, Vickers AJ, Joffe E, et al. **Prostate Cancer Foundation Screening Guidelines for Black Men in the United States.** *NEJM Evid.* 2024;3(4). doi:10.1056/EVIDoa2300289

32. American Diabetes Association. **2. Classification and Diagnosis of Diabetes: Standards of Care in Diabetes—2024.** *Diabetes Care.* 2024;47(Suppl 1):S16–S38. doi:10.2337/dc24-S002

33. Machalek DA, Grulich AE, Jin F, et al. **Anal Human Papillomavirus Infection and Associated Neoplasia in Men Who Have Sex with Men: A Systematic Review and Meta-analysis.** *Lancet Oncol.* 2012;13(5):487–500. doi:10.1016/S1470-2045(12)70080-3

34. CDC. **Recommended Adult Immunization Schedule: United States, 2024.** Advisory Committee on Immunization Practices (ACIP). Available at: https://www.cdc.gov/vaccines/schedules/hcp/adult.html

35. Schillie S, Wester C, Osborne M, Wesolowski L, Ryerson AB. **CDC Recommendations for Hepatitis C Screening Among Adults—United States, 2020.** *MMWR Recomm Rep.* 2020;69(2):1–17.

36. American Diabetes Association. **11. Chronic Kidney Disease and Risk Management: Standards of Care in Diabetes—2024.** *Diabetes Care.* 2024;47(Suppl 1):S191–S202. doi:10.2337/dc24-S011

37. Palefsky JM, Giuliano AR, Goldstone S, et al. **Anal Human Papillomavirus Infection and Anal Intraepithelial Neoplasia in HIV-Positive Men and Women.** *J Infect Dis.* 2011;203(3):286–295. doi:10.1093/infdis/jiq053

38. D'Souza G, Wiley DJ, Li X, et al. **Incidence and Epidemiology of Anal Cancer in the Multicenter AIDS Cohort Study.** *J Acquir Immune Defic Syndr.* 2008;48(4):491–499. doi:10.1097/QAI.0b013e31817aebfe

39. Silverberg MJ, Lau B, Achenbach CJ, et al. **Cumulative Incidence of Cancer Among Persons With HIV in North America: A Cohort Study.** *Ann Intern Med.* 2015;163(7):507–518. doi:10.7326/M14-2768

40. Panel on Opportunistic Infections in Adults and Adolescents with HIV. **Guidelines for the Prevention and Treatment of Opportunistic Infections in Adults and Adolescents with HIV: Human Papillomavirus Disease.** Department of Health and Human Services. 2023.

BIBLIOGRAPHY

41. Palefsky JM. **Practicing high-resolution anoscopy.** *Curr Opin Oncol.* 2009;21(5):482-486. doi:10.1097/CCO.0b013e32832e0cdb
42. Panel on Opportunistic Infections. **Hepatitis B Virus Infection.** ClinicalInfo.HIV.gov. 2023. Accessed April 14, 2025. https://clinicalinfo.hiv.gov/en/guidelines
43. Centers for Disease Control and Prevention. **Latent TB Infection Testing and Diagnosis.** Updated 2022. https://www.cdc.gov/tb/topic/testing/
44. Workowski KA, Bachmann LH, Chan PA, et al. **Sexually transmitted infections treatment guidelines, 2021.** *MMWR Recomm Rep.* 2021;70(4):1-187.
45. Mbaeyi SA, Bozio CH, Dooling KL. **Updated recommendations for use of pneumococcal vaccines in adults.** *MMWR Morb Mortal Wkly Rep.* 2022;71(4):109-117.
46. Thornhill JP, Barkati S, Walmsley S, et al. **Monkeypox virus infection in humans across 16 countries — April–June 2022.** *N Engl J Med.* 2022;387(8):679-691.
47. Baden LR, El Sahly HM, Essink B, et al. **Efficacy and safety of the mRNA-1273 SARS-CoV-2 vaccine.** *N Engl J Med.* 2021;384(5):403-416.
48. Grohskopf LA, Alyanak E, Ferdinands JM, et al. **Prevention and control of seasonal influenza with vaccines: Recommendations of the ACIP—United States, 2023–24.** *MMWR Recomm Rep.* 2023;72(1):1-28.
49. Panel on Guidelines for the Prevention and Treatment of Opportunistic Infections in Adults and Adolescents with HIV. **Human papillomavirus disease.** Clinicalinfo.HIV.gov. Updated July 9, 2024. Accessed February 24, 2025. https://clinicalinfo.hiv.gov/en/guidelines/hiv-clinical-guidelines-adult-and-adolescent-opportunistic-infections/human?view=full
50. Centers for Disease Control and Prevention. **Clinical guidelines on the use of doxycycline postexposure prophylaxis for bacterial STI prevention.** MMWR Recomm Rep. 2024;73(2): 1-16.
51. Molina JM, Charreau I, Chidiac C, et al. **Postexposure doxycycline to prevent bacterial sexually transmitted infections.** N Engl J Med. 2023;388(14):1296-1306. doi:10.1056/NEJMoa2211934

BIBLIOGRAPHY

52. Luetkemeyer AF, Donnell D, Dombrowski JC, et al. **Doxycycline postexposure prophylaxis for bacterial sexually transmitted infections.** N Engl J Med. 2023;388(14):1296-1306. doi:10.1056/NEJMoa2211934

53. Volk JE, Marcus JL, Phengrasamy T, et al. **Doxycycline postexposure prophylaxis for bacterial sexually transmitted infections among men who have sex with men: a randomized controlled trial.** JAMA Intern Med. 2024;184(3):1-9. doi:10.1001/jamainternmed.2024.1234

www.ingramcontent.com/pod-product-compliance
Lightning Source LLC
Chambersburg PA
CBHW020553030426
42337CB00013B/1078